Reaching for Answers to Crohn's Disease

Reaching for Answers to Crohn's Disease

*A Story of Success with Diet and Probiotics
as Recommended by J. Rainer Poley, M.D.*

Martha Kalichman, R.N.

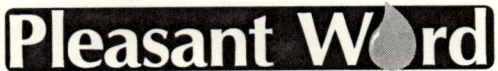

© 2008 by Martha Kalichman. All rights reserved.

Cover photo by Kelly Brewer

Pleasant Word (a division of WinePress Publishing, PO Box 428, Enumclaw, WA 98022) functions only as book publisher. As such, the ultimate design, content, editorial accuracy, and views expressed or implied in this work are those of the author.

No part of this publication may be reproduced, stored in a retrieval system, or transmitted in any way by any means—electronic, mechanical, photocopy, recording, or otherwise—without the prior permission of the copyright holder, except as provided by USA copyright law.

The author of this book has waived the publisher's suggested editing services. As such, the author is responsible for any errors found in this finished product.

Unless otherwise noted, all Scriptures are taken from the *Holy Bible, New International Version®, NIV®*. Copyright © 1973, 1978, 1984 by the International Bible Society. Used by permission of Zondervan. All rights reserved.

ISBN 13: 978-1-4141-1176-6
ISBN 10: 1-4141-1176-2
Library of Congress Catalog Card Number: 2008900116

This book is dedicated to my mother,
Marjorie, who instilled
in me the joy of writing and the benefits of
keeping a journal.

The suggestions contained in this book are not intended as a substitute for medical treatment by a physician. They reflect the author's experiences, research, and opinions. Neither the author nor the publisher is responsible for any adverse effects or consequences from the use of information presented in this book.

Contents

Acknowledgments xi
Introduction xiii

1. Low Grade and Rising.................. 1
2. Orange Teeth......................... 7
3. Waiting for Answers 11
4. A Piece of Cake......................15
5. Just Believe 19
6. Piercing Words 23
7. Go Home and Eat Some Bugs 27
8. Write It on the Calendar 33
9. The Amazing Journey 35
10. Simple Answers......................39

11. Where the Bugs Reign 43
12. Friendly Bacteria 49
13. Enjoy Life 55
14. Diet Guidelines 57

Recipes 63
Endnotes 81
References 85

Acknowledgments

As I sit in the empty bedroom of my daughter, Sarah, who is now away at college, the butterflies painted on her walls remind me of the freedom from illness she enjoys. Four years ago she began a journey of breaking the cocoon-like restraints that Crohn's disease placed on her. Today I feel overwhelming appreciation to many who have traveled this path of change with us and have assisted me in telling our story.

I have enormous gratitude to Dr. J. Rainer Poley, who changed the course of my daughter's life through his willingness to treat her with a sucrose-restricted diet and probiotics.

I am grateful for Sarah's compliance in following Dr. Poley's instructions. Without her cooperation and discipline, this story of hope to share with others would not exist.

I am grateful for my husband Michael's commitment to explore with me a different route as we sought help for our daughter.

The assistance and encouragement of Sarah, Michael, and Dr. Poley have enabled me to write this book. My profound thankfulness also goes to Barbara Baranowski and Kay Walsh for their never ending patience, advice, and support in pursuing this venture. In addition, I want to thank the members of the writer's group I attend (Richmond Christians Who Write), and also Nancy Farrar, who have helped me with this endeavor.

Most importantly, I would like to express my deepest gratitude to the Lord for restoring my daughter's health by revealing His clear direction to us as Sarah battled Crohn's disease and won. He is the true Author of this story and the freedom she possesses.

Introduction

Many times, listening to stories from others fighting the battle against Crohn's disease has deeply touched my heart. One night a friend called, asking me to visit a patient she cared for who suffered with this disease. "I've tried explaining to her the diet that Sarah is following," she said, "but I think it would be helpful if you would talk to her."

The next day, as I approached the elevator in the hospital, memories of my own fears flooded my mind. Several years earlier our daughter, Sarah, had been diagnosed with Crohn's disease. At that time I had wondered if she would ever have to confront intestinal surgery.

When I visited the young lady, her pale color indicated the reason for the unit of blood hanging beside her bed. She was facing surgery the next day to remove a portion of her intestine damaged by Crohn's disease. Following doctor's orders, she had taken numerous medications every day for years, but still intestinal damage prevailed. When I left her room, my mind was consumed by the thought: *Maybe life could have been different for her if she had only known about the treatment Sarah is following.* Therefore, my passion to tell others about our personal experience continues.

As I write this, Sarah has been in remission of Crohn's disease for over four years, by following the instructions of her pediatric gastroenterologist, Dr. J. Rainer Poley. Based on his research and knowledge, he recommended that she follow a sucrose-restricted diet, eat plain yogurt, and take probiotics. The purpose of the sucrose-restricted diet is to "starve" the harmful bacteria by removing their major food source. Consuming yogurt and probiotics helps replenish the "good" bacteria, therefore, resulting in a balance of the intestinal bacteria. Studies done in past medical research that provide the rationale for following this treatment will be discussed in future chapters. Thus, through my writing and sharing this information I hope to positively affect the lives of others.

Martha Kalichman

Chapter 1

Low Grade and Rising

"Goodnight, Sarah. See you in the morning," I said as I gave my fifteen-year-old daughter a hug. "Gosh, you sure feel warm. Maybe we should check your temperature."

"Oh, Mom," she said as she rolled her eyes.

Sarah and her older brother, Josh, have sometimes felt plagued by having parents who are both registered nurses. Although my husband, Michael, switched careers years ago, we have always been attuned to any symptoms of ill health that our children often wished we would ignore.

"This will only take a minute," I said as I got the thermometer. Sure enough, the mercury climbed, indicating a low-grade fever. Earlier that day Sarah had received her allergy shot, so I presumed it was the culprit.

The fever lingered into the next day, prompting me to call the allergist. As reported by his nurse, the doctor responded that it was rare to have a fever from an allergy shot. He thought Sarah probably had a cold virus.

However, after the next allergy shot a week later, the fever returned. Once again the allergist assumed a virus had caused it. He instructed us to consult the pediatrician if Sarah had further problems.

The following morning, Sarah began a summer physical education class. When I picked her up from school later that day, she reported she had felt lightheaded after participating in outdoor activities. Then, she asked a question that would be etched in my mind for the next year: "Mom, what do you think is wrong with me?"

"Maybe you just need to drink more water when you're outside in the heat," I replied. With temperatures in the upper 90s, the dog days of summer had definitely arrived.

Later that afternoon, Sarah's temperature once again began to rise. Since she complained of a headache, I took her to the pediatrician. He suspected the beginning of a sinus infection and ordered lab work. Sarah had the tests, and we went home, awaiting the results.

Before I answered the phone on Saturday morning, I noticed the doctor's name on the caller ID. I feared the worst, because doctors usually don't call on weekends. He reported that Sarah's lab work showed a hemoglobin of 10.

"It's probably only iron deficiency anemia, so I would like her to take an iron supplement," the pediatrician said. Many times in the recent past we had blamed her frequent complaints of fatigue on her allergies, but obviously, anemia contributed to this problem. Since the pediatrician also surmised that a sinus infection was a possibility, he ordered an antibiotic. Nevertheless, he felt she could continue her physical education class.

Sarah began taking an iron supplement and the prescribed antibiotic. She struggled to keep up with the other students. Watching her battle exhaustion gripped my heart, but I could not persuade Sarah to drop the class. Her determination, along with the doctor's approval to press on, overruled me. The five weeks of that class seemed like five months. I dropped Sarah off at school each day early in the morning and went home and prayed. Gradually her energy level increased, and she successfully finished the course.

A month later Sarah's allergist suggested that she resume her regular shots. I felt hesitant about subjecting her to more injections but agreed to give it one more try. Later in the day, after she had received the shots, Sarah complained about feeling warm. The low-grade fever had returned. The following morning I called the allergist, and we agreed that Sarah should not receive any more allergy shots. We hoped no further side effects would result from the recent injections.

However, two days before an upcoming summer retreat, the fever lingered. Sarah asked, "Can I still go to the youth retreat?"

"We'll just have to wait to see how you're feeling," I said.

We waited until the last minute to make a decision, hoping that somehow we would know for sure if she should go. Although she had anticipated the four-day youth retreat for weeks, I wondered if she could physically handle it. I knew the days would be packed with activities, morning to night, with limited sleeping time.

"Let's check your temperature one more time," I said.

It was 99.8. Would her temperature rise as it had the past several evenings? Would she get worse if I let her go? She was in tears while we discussed it.

"Oh, Lord, what should she do?" I silently prayed.

Looking up, I noticed the screen saver message moving across our computer screen. I had read it many times, but at that moment the message was clear: "Don't be afraid, just believe" (Luke 8:50).

    I turned to Sarah and gave her a hug. "You can go," I said. The words on the computer screen had relieved my fear. Sarah had a great time, and the fever was totally gone when she returned home from the retreat. This lesson of trust helped prepare my husband and me for the journey ahead in the coming year.

Chapter 2

Orange Teeth

Sarah began her sophomore year of high school feeling well and more energetic than she had been in the summertime. Thus, we assumed the doctor had made the right diagnosis: "just iron deficiency anemia," although other issues began to arise.

"Even my friends think my teeth look orange!" Sarah exclaimed one day when she came home from school.

"Let me see," I said earnestly as she opened her mouth.

Her dad looked, too. "They do look a little orange."

The week before, I had noticed her teeth exhibiting a glimmer of orange tint but didn't think about it any further. Now her friends were noticing. Wondering if she had taken the iron tablets too long, I called her doctor.

Since recent lab work showed that her iron levels still lingered below normal, the doctor wanted Sarah to continue taking iron supplements. "Our bodies tend to get rid of any extra iron," he said. "The orange color probably comes from plaque on Sarah's teeth."

However, knowing her diligence in brushing and flossing, I decided to call the dentist for his opinion. He had observed children with orange-tinted teeth who live in areas with high iron content in the water. Excess iron in their saliva evidently caused the discoloration. The dentist stressed that no physical harm would come from this condition, and he advised us to follow the pediatrician's instructions. But the emotional drain caused by peer ridicule concerned me. What teenager wants to have orange teeth? Temporarily, we decreased the iron supplements; in a couple of weeks, Sarah's teeth resumed a normal color.

Another trip to the lab several months later revealed a normal hemoglobin level, but Sarah's red blood cell size remained abnormally small. This finding indicated that her body still lacked proper absorption of the iron supplements. Furthermore, Sarah's energy level continued to drag.

It was heartbreaking to notice her refraining from participation in activities with friends. Although she worked diligently, keeping up with school work became harder. Lab tests became a familiar event, and concern that a condition more serious than iron deficiency anemia existed necessitated a referral to a specialist.

Chapter 3

Waiting for Answers

The echoes of our footsteps bounced off the walls of the long corridor that led us to the office of the pediatric hematologist. Surreal thoughts filled my mind while Sarah, Michael, and I sat in the waiting room amid young, bald-headed children. As they played video games, they seemed oblivious to the serious conditions that I presumed they faced. I wondered how the parents dealt with their children's illnesses.

Our time in this room seemed interminable to me, but Sarah enjoyed playing a game from the countless selections. The nurse assured us that the highly recommended doctor was worth the wait, and when we finally met the physician, we realized the truth in her words. She thoroughly examined Sarah and ordered more lab tests. By her calm nature and compassion, we felt reassured.

After spending the entire afternoon in the office, Sarah exclaimed on our way out, "That was the best doctor's appointment I've ever had!" Large, fluffy snowflakes greeted us at the door. They softly touched our faces and gently fell on our shoulders as we walked to the car. We had no new answers, but the quietness and beauty of the snow-filled air filtered the turmoil from our thoughts.

We felt relieved several weeks later to learn that Sarah did not have a terminal illness. Although some of the lab tests were normal, others needed to be repeated due to incorrect labeling. Getting Sarah out of school for the afternoon and making another trip to the hospital discouraged both of us, as we realized this would be yet an additional delay in determining a diagnosis.

Another two weeks passed before we received the normal lab results. Even though that news brought some relief to us, our impatience to find the cause of Sarah's anemia grew. Suspecting a malabsorption problem, the hematologist referred her to a gastroenterologist.

While Sarah and I rode to the doctor's office for an appointment with the specialist, we had high hopes of gaining some clue to the problem. Michael left work to meet us. During our time spent in the waiting room, I picked up one of the doctor's business cards from the counter. Numerous titles followed his name, so I thought surely this doctor would find the missing piece of the puzzle.

The nurse called us back to an examination room. When the doctor entered the room, he appeared rushed and impatiently listened to our questions. Quickly he examined Sarah and ordered an upper gastrointestinal series of x-rays. Sarah, Michael, and I left the office with great disappointment. Michael returned to work; I took Sarah back to school, and then I drove home and cried. Frustration flooded my mind, as the hope of soon finding the answer to Sarah's problem faded.

Since clear, caring communication is a priority to us during doctor appointments, we felt the need to seek out another physician. A friend suggested one who might be able to help us determine the next step. A few phone calls later, our hope revived when we received a referral to another gastroenterologist.

Chapter 4

A Piece of Cake

As we anticipated the upper gastrointestinal test that Sarah faced, we heard many negative comments about drinking the barium liquid for this x-ray. Finally, the day before the scheduled test, a friend shared encouraging words. "I had that test done last year. It was a piece of cake," she said. "Actually I thought the barium drink tasted pretty good. It didn't bother me at all!" What peace her words gave me. I could hardly wait to tell Sarah when she came home from school that day.

Early the next morning, Michael and I took Sarah for the x-rays. The nurse handed her a cup of barium to drink, along with a cup of another liquid. Sarah came out in the hallway to sit with us while she drank it. "It tastes pretty good—kind of a tropical flavor," she said.

I had to laugh. "I guess my friend was right." The rest of the procedure went well, too—"a piece of cake."

Afterwards, the radiologist came from the x-ray room to tell us the results. "I have good news and bad news. The good news is Sarah doesn't have Crohn's disease; the bad news is we don't know why she's anemic." Truly, it was great news to hear that Sarah did not have Crohn's disease, but what was wrong?

On the ride home Sarah asked, "Do you think I could go back to school? If we get there by 2:30, I could still go to the last class, and then I wouldn't be counted absent for the day." She had received many awards in the past but never one for perfect attendance. Even through all of this, she wanted to try.

Her dad and I looked at each other, not knowing what to say. "Are you sure you feel up to it?" Michael asked.

"Yes, I feel fine," she insisted. Persuaded by her plea, we drove to the school.

"What an amazing day! Never would I have imagined we'd be bringing her to school today," I said to Michael as we watched Sarah walk through the school doors. He agreed.

At the end of that school year, we attended the annual awards ceremony. Michael and I knew how hard the year had been for Sarah. She would awaken in the morning feeling tired before the day started. Then, she would come home after school with even greater fatigue, yet strive to get her schoolwork done. While we both tried to suppress the tears, we watched her receive several awards for outstanding academic achievement and even a perfect attendance award.

Chapter 5

Just Believe

Although the upper GI series of x-rays revealed no problems, further testing was still needed to determine if Sarah had a malabsorption disorder. When we saw the gastroenterologist, he ordered a colonoscopy. We decided to postpone it until after our family vacation. Since we had already waited a year for a diagnosis, what harm would there be in waiting two more weeks? We had planned to visit Laura Ingalls Wilder's home in Missouri, because the stories in her books had touched all of our lives from our children's earliest years. At last, we were able to fit the trip into our summer plans. Fortunately, Sarah seemed to be feeling fine.

As we toured Wilder's home, Michael and I remembered with fondness reading her stories to

Sarah and Josh during their childhood. The tall trees towering over Wilder's house and the summer sounds in the countryside brought the peace I longed for. A small inn located in the nearby town seemed like a perfect place to spend the night. We welcomed the slower pace of life, and for a brief time, the thought of Sarah's problems drifted away.

However, early the next morning, Sarah awoke not feeling well. After repeatedly vomiting, she fell back to sleep, along with everyone else in the family except me. I tried to act calm on the outside, but my heart was pounding. We were many miles away from home. I went outside to sit in the car to read, but thoughts bombarded my mind. What was wrong with Sarah? And then it dawned on me—Sarah usually drank only distilled water. We had discovered when she was two-years old that continually drinking tap water upset her stomach. We never knew why, but it definitely caused distress. I suddenly realized she had been drinking tap water frequently over the past two days. She had brought several bottles of distilled water on the trip, but we had neglected to replenish the supply. I immediately went to the local store to buy more water.

Amazingly, several hours later, Sarah felt better. We were able to spend the rest of the day at Wilder's house and then continue our travel plans.

Our travels took us through the beautiful landscape of the Midwest to areas we had never seen. Sarah felt fine for several days, and then one morning she awoke not feeling well. Fear gripped me once again. *Maybe we shouldn't have waited two more weeks for the colonoscopy; maybe she is sicker than we thought.*

Sarah and Michael soon fell back asleep, but Josh and I decided to eat breakfast. When we crept quietly to the door, I noticed Sarah's Bible on the edge of the table. I picked it up as we walked out of the room. While the two of us sat in the dining room, I found tucked in Sarah's Bible an index card with Scriptures she had written. As I went down the list, I came to Luke 8:50: "Don't be afraid; just believe, and she will be healed." These were the words that I noticed on the computer screen the summer before, except the phrase "she will be healed" had not been included. Peace came over me. When we went back to the room, Sarah was better, so we continued our vacation. The rest of our travels went fine, and Sarah felt well.

Chapter 6

Piercing Words

After we returned home, Sarah had the scheduled colonoscopy. "I am almost one-hundred percent sure your daughter has Crohn's disease," the doctor told Michael and me while Sarah was still in recovery. The words pierced my heart. I wanted to deny the diagnosis, but knew I needed to accept it. However, peace eluded me even further when I learned of the strong medications the doctor wanted Sarah to start taking. As a nurse, I knew the risk of detrimental, long-term side effects of the drugs prescribed for Crohn's disease.

When I asked the doctor if diet had anything to do with Crohn's disease, he said it did not, but that Sarah should avoid eating nuts and popcorn, which are hard to digest. Although I knew that many in the medical community categorized Crohn's disease as an autoimmune disorder, it seemed odd that diet would have so little to do with a gastrointestinal problem. Therefore, I decided to research that issue. The next day while searching the internet, I learned of the book *Breaking the Vicious Cycle* by Elaine Gottschall. I promptly purchased a copy from a nearby bookstore, began skimming through it, and read about the diet the author promoted. It seemed rigid and hard to follow. At that point I just wanted to escape from the problem for a few days. I was too weary to change anything until we knew a definite diagnosis from the colonoscopy biopsy report.

The next day I remembered a story my mother had told me months before. A friend of hers had a granddaughter who had been diagnosed with Crohn's disease several years before and recently had learned she had been misdiagnosed. When I later talked to the mother of this girl, she strongly suggested we get another opinion. I appreciated her suggestion, although I didn't have any idea whom we would see for another opinion.

That afternoon as I was fixing dinner, a storm knocked out our electricity. While I waited for it to return, I picked up the book by Elaine Gottschall and started reading it from the beginning. When I got to page eight, it was obvious a different Power was at work as I read the name Dr. J. Rainer Poley.

He had conducted extensive research on the effect of certain sugars and starches on people with intestinal diseases. The author of the book had cited the name *Eastern Virginia Medical School* in her reference about this doctor. Almost in disbelief, I reread the school's name; it was located only two hours from us. I quickly looked up Dr. Poley's phone number and learned that he was in practice as a pediatric gastroenterologist. His office was at a large children's hospital affiliated with the nursing school I had graduated from years ago. When Michael came home from work, I shared what I had read about Dr. Poley. We both knew without a doubt that we wanted Sarah to see this doctor for a third opinion.

Chapter 7

Go Home and Eat Some Bugs

When we saw Dr. Poley, he thoroughly examined Sarah and reviewed her medical history. He proved to be kind and genuinely interested. Since Sarah only had occasional gastrointestinal symptoms, the *IBD-First Step* lab test was ordered to confirm the Crohn's disease diagnosis from the colonoscopy report. This test has a fairly high incidence of accuracy in identifying antibodies which are elevated in Crohn's disease and ulcerative colitis. I felt relieved that he comprehensively searched for an accurate diagnosis.

Two weeks later we went for Sarah's next doctor's appointment. The results of the lab test strongly indicated that she did indeed have Crohn's disease. We asked him if there was any other treatment Sarah could try besides medications. He explained that at a medical conference in Europe that summer, he had learned of success medical doctors were having with probiotics. He instructed Sarah to eat plain yogurt every day and to take a specific probiotic capsule called Culturelle® containing the Lactobacillus GG bacteria strain twice daily. Based on his research, he wanted Sarah to limit her consumption of concentrated sugars (specifically table sugar, technically known as sucrose). According to Dr. Poley, it has been well documented that "sucrose is the prime energy source for commensal bacteria, which seem responsible for triggering the inflammatory process in Crohn's disease." The intent of the sucrose-restricted diet was to starve the harmful bacteria by taking away their major food source. The yogurt and Lactobacillus GG would help replenish the "good" bacteria.

At the conclusion of our appointment, he looked at Sarah and kindly said with a smile, "So, go home and eat some bugs." We all laughed, feeling hopeful that these "bugs" would help.

On our way home we bought some plain yogurt. I had not eaten plain yogurt before, but now I became acutely aware of how much sugar those tempting flavored ones contain. I wanted to support Sarah in her new diet, so we both sat at the table with our bowls of yogurt. After I took one spoonful, I looked up and said, "Maybe some fruit will help."

"Maybe so," she said.

After adding some sliced grapes and strawberries, we both agreed the fruit made a big difference! Eventually, Sarah enjoyed eating it without adding fruit.

We began reading food labels in our pantry, pulling out any foods that had more than three grams of added sugar per serving and placing them elsewhere. I hoped that "out of sight, out of mind" would help her resist the tempting snacks.

A few days before Sarah began her junior year in high school, we saw one of her favorite teachers from the previous year. Whenever Sarah needed to get lab work done during her sophomore year, she usually missed part of her late afternoon chemistry class. Therefore, the teacher became aware of Sarah's health problem. She had shown genuine concern and care for Sarah throughout that year. As we chatted with her, we told her about the doctor we had found two hours away and the instructions Sarah was following. Since this teacher had once worked at Eastern Virginia Medical School, she inquired about the doctor's name. We told her, and to our surprise, we learned she had worked in the electron microscopy lab for Dr. Poley years before. She spoke highly of him. Her encouraging words confirmed that we were truly on the right path.

Two weeks later, Sarah began to feel better in general. By the end of the first month, she had gained two pounds, which was significant since she had not gained any weight during the previous eighteen months. Her endurance increased, and she began feeling well consistently, every day. At the follow-up appointment with Dr. Poley three months later, he thought Sarah looked healthy and hoped that her lab work would confirm that.

The day before we were to find out the lab results, doubt began to cloud my thoughts. Were the probiotics and diet helping Sarah enough to bring her lab work up to normal? I knew her doctor wanted it to work too, but if it didn't, I assumed he would need to place Sarah on medications. I had seen the Lord's hand in so many details of this journey, but fear tried to undermine my hope. I went for a walk late in the afternoon that day and poured out my heart.

> *Dear Lord,*
> *There is a part of me that feels You are healing Sarah, and yet I'm afraid to trust that thought. We have been on this journey for so long. I yearn for Your light of hope to shine on the path ahead. There are still rocks that cause me to stumble—to fall into a thicket of*

doubt. I feel entrapped by fear that Sarah will not be well. Your words have reminded me repeatedly to fear not—but just believe, and yet I continually need reassurance. Please forgive me for doubting, and help me to trust You and believe Your promises.

Amen.

As I walked back to the house, I was ready to relinquish my worries, for only then was there room for me to accept His peace. The turmoil that had raced through my mind earlier dissolved.

The next day when Dr. Poley called, my heart stood still, knowing that the news he was about to share would be crucial in our lives. "I want to report that Sarah's lab results are all normal!" he said. He gave instructions for her to continue the same regimen and to return in four months for a follow-up visit and lab work. I thanked him profusely for calling and could hardly contain my elation!

After I got off the phone, I ran to Sarah and Michael with the news. We all hugged each other as we truly experienced the joy of answered prayers!

Chapter 8

Write It on the Calendar

We felt grateful to have found a doctor who prescribed a treatment that restored Sarah's health without powerful drugs. Unfortunately, after the second visit with Dr. Poley, we learned he was planning to relocate to another area. "I'll let you know more when plans are definite," he said.

Since he had advised us to return in four months for lab work to make sure that the diet and probiotics were continuing to resolve the problem, we made an appointment with another doctor for April 14th. However, we decided we wanted Sarah to continue seeing Dr. Poley if we could make the trip in a day. Two months, then three passed. In April, there were still no firm plans in place.

Several days before the April 14th appointment, I was sharing my frustrations with a friend during a phone conversation. "It sure seems like I can count on answers to prayer to be revealed at the last minute," I joked. "The last possible date that we could cancel the April 14th appointment with the other doctor would be April 13th. Maybe I should just write it on the calendar that on April 13th Dr. Poley will call." We both laughed.

April 13th arrived, and Sarah informed me before she went to school that morning that it was important for her not to miss the next day of school. "Could we just reschedule the appointment for another time?" she asked. Sarah was continuing to feel well, so I agreed and made the phone call.

Later that day, as though I really could have marked it on my calendar, Dr. Poley called! Plans were now definite that he would be in practice at a medical school that was three hours from where we lived. After I hung up the phone, I laughed out loud and called my husband at work, and we laughed some more.

Sarah has continued to see Dr. Poley for the past four years for follow-up visits. We feel grateful that she remains in remission, with normal lab results, as well as normal physical examinations.

Chapter 9

The Amazing Journey

As a nurse, I realize the importance of having basic knowledge about the digestion process when trying to understand how diet and probiotics affect intestinal health. Most of us give little thought of what happens to a morsel of food once it passes our taste buds. However, it encounters an amazing journey, starting from the mouth, traveling down the esophagus and into the stomach, through many feet of the small and large intestines, until it is excreted from the body.

When the food reaches the stomach it encounters powerful gastric juices. In 1822, physician William Beaumont had the opportunity to study gastric juices and their functions when he treated a man who was accidentally shot in the stomach.[1] After the wound healed, a permanent opening was left. He often has been referred to as the "man with a window in his stomach." This hole enabled Beaumont to observe the changes in the stomach and explain digestion as a chemical process.

In this process, by the time the food has been churned and mixed with gastric juices in the stomach, it turns into a thick liquid called *chyme*. It then flows into the small intestine, which is divided into three sections. The first ten inches of the small intestine is called the *duodenum,* followed by a section about ten feet long called the *jejunum,* which extends into the ileum, the remaining ten feet of the small intestine.

Located on the mucous membrane lining of the small intestine are finger-like projections called *villi* and *microvilli*, which absorb the nutrients as the chyme travels along the digestive tract. The intestinal mucous membrane is armed to block out any foreign substances attempting to invade the body. When the nutrients have been absorbed, they pass into the small blood vessels, which transport them to the liver.

After the small intestine has assimilated all the nutrients, any food remaining that is not digested or absorbed travels through a valve connecting the small intestine to the large intestine. This valve prevents the waste from returning into the small intestine. The four to five feet of the large intestine consists of sections called the *cecum*, the *colon*, the *rectum*, and the *anal canal*, where the waste leaves the body.

Depending on the population of commensal bacteria and its effects on the immune system, clinical symptoms of inflammatory bowel disease (IBD) may vary widely. Many affect the digestive tract, including diarrhea, nausea, vomiting, fatigue, and abdominal pain, which can be vague or intense, especially on the right, lower side where the small and large intestines connect at the end of the ileum. Fever, bleeding, anemia, mouth ulcers, and constipation can also occur. Symptoms outside of the intestinal system, such as arthritis, joint pain, fistulas, and eczema, may develop. These clinical symptoms indicate the need for various tests to determine a definite diagnosis.

Blood tests and stool cultures are helpful in establishing a diagnosis of IBD (Crohn's disease or ulcerative colitis). A complete blood count (CBC) is done to determine if there is a low hemoglobin or hematocrit level due to iron deficiency from malabsorption or blood loss. The size of the red blood cells is indicated by the Mean Corpuscular Volume (MCV). If a lack of iron absorption exists, these cells may be abnormally small. Erythrocyte sedimentation rate (sed rate) and C-reactive protein

(CRP) tests verify if an inflammatory process persists somewhere in the body, although they are not specific to location. Low albumin levels due to increased intestinal protein loss caused by the inflammatory process may occur. Stool cultures are done and can reveal a hidden blood loss. All of these tests help to assess the necessity for further tests.

If suspicion of inflammatory bowel disease continues, evaluation by an upper and lower endoscopy becomes essential. Since the results of biopsy reports done during these tests sometimes reveal inconclusive results, the *IBD-First Step* blood test, later replaced by the newer, more accurate version of *Prometheus® IBD serology 7*, provides benefits in confirming a questionable diagnosis of IBD. This test identifies antibody markers that usually are elevated in Crohn's disease or ulcerative colitis.

Thus, the health of the digestive tract influences complete health, and the effects of diseases are revealed through medical tests. An understanding of the digestive process and its reactions gives insight into more effective care.

Chapter 10

Simple Answers

Questions lingered in my mind about intestinal diseases. When the gastroenterologist who did the colonoscopy diagnosed Sarah with Crohn's disease, my initial intuitive questions centered on the effects diet has on this disease. The doctor's answer focused on medications, seemingly a common focus for the majority of the medical community.

While searching for articles during one of my visits to a local medical library, a revealing thought permeated my mind: *countless answers to medical questions from previous years fill the pages of books in these rooms.* As I walked down aisle after aisle amid rows of shelves containing volumes of medical research, I realized I could not comprehend the vastness of the knowledge they disclosed. An awareness infiltrated my thoughts that although there are many brilliant doctors, the human mind cannot possibly learn all that has been researched even in one specialty. Yet, from the knowledge, research, and experience of our daughter's doctor, he provided her with the unique, simple dietary and probiotic treatment that restored her health.

Crohn's disease is currently viewed as a disorder that cannot be cured. Many people suffering with this disease are robbed of good health for years. Some are brought into remission through medications or surgery, but the risk of long-term ill effects from these treatments is a reality.

Researchers have attempted to unveil the mystery of inflammatory bowel disease for many years. The intricate complexities of Crohn's disease still are not understood fully, and the persistent search for the missing puzzle pieces continues. However, preliminary scientific evidence has revealed clues to the credibility of the treatment that initiated the continued remission of Crohn's disease for Sarah and others.

The following sections address some of the research that affirms the plausibility of the regimen Sarah follows. While there have been studies done on the effects of a restricted-sugar diet and the effects of probiotics, research that combines the two approaches is lacking. These studies lead to the conclusion that the prospect of a sucrose-restricted diet and the use of a reliable probiotic such as Culturelle®, which contains Lactobacillus GG bacteria, could benefit many people suffering with Crohn's disease.

Chapter 11

Where the Bugs Reign

Up until birth, there are no bacteria in the human gastrointestinal tract, but from the moment a baby enters the world, the bacteria from the environment begin to colonize in the baby's intestinal tract. Much past research helps us understand the important role of these bacteria.

Prior to the Apollo trip to the moon in the 1970s, no one knew what types of bacteria the astronauts could feasibly transport back to the earth. A complete identification of the many existing bacteria types in the intestinal tract had not been done, thus creating the need for in-depth research.[1] The research of Moore, Holdeman, and colleagues at Virginia Polytechnic Institute was the first to identify and describe the multiple species of bacteria thriving in the colon.[2] These 400 to 500 species of bacteria are commonly referred to as *microflora*, or *flora*.[1, 2] Through the years, researchers have continued to study intestinal flora.

The bacteria that live in the human digestive system help maintain normal intestinal health by protecting the body from disease-producing bacteria called *pathogens*. Some of the bacteria in the intestinal tract maintain a stable population, and some ingested bacteria simply flow through, possibly containing pathogens.[1] Due to the hydrochloric acid in the stomach, many bacteria cannot survive, dying as they leave the stomach and travel to the small intestine.[1] Under normal conditions, the majority of the organisms in the intestines, also often referred to as the gut, are harmless and live together in harmony. But an imbalance may occur.

Although the cause for the initiation and progression of inflammatory bowel disease remains unknown, much evidence indicates that an overgrowth of bacteria contributes a significant role in the development of IBD. It is commonly agreed that the immune system is acting in response to the microflora that inhabit the gastrointestinal tract; however, the trigger for the onset of this action is not clear.[3] It may be attributed to an abundance of either normal or disease-producing bacteria.[4] As summarized by Dr. Poley, "Two mutations of a gene called *NOD2/CARD 15* on chromosome 16 provide the genetic liability to develop Crohn's disease, mainly of the terminal ileum. Mutations in certain parts of this gene do not make possible certain defense mechanisms and help the production of an inflammatory response." This discovery shows a connection between bacteria and an inflammatory process in the digestive tract.[5]

In J. R. Poley's research on fifty-six children who suffered from varying types of chronic diarrhea, biopsies were taken from the duodeno-jejunal junction, which is the link between the first two sections of the small intestine.[6] Typically in healthy people that area of the small intestine has either no microorganisms or an insignificant number, but one of Poley's major findings revealed increased bacterial activity from that area. He also noted a presence of excessive mucus, causing a barrier along the intestinal mucosa and, therefore, inhibiting the absorption of some nutrients. The cause of the increased mucus may be due to increased bacterial activity and the presence of bacterial toxins.[6] The small intestine provides the most important location for digestion and absorption of nutrients, so if a barrier of mucus prevents the digestion of nutrients, the body does not receive the fuel it needs to function properly.

Nevertheless, diet can affect the overgrowth of intestinal flora that may be precipitating the increased mucus, causing a barrier and preventing the absorption of nutrients.[6] Since "sucrose serves as a prime energy source for commensal bacteria in the intestinal tract," as stated by Dr. Poley, he recommends a sucrose-restricted diet to promote an environment where much of the bacterial overgrowth will lose the food supply and "starve."

Other research on diet and Crohn's disease has been conducted. In 1984 Ó'Moráin and colleagues found that an elemental diet, a liquid diet containing all the necessary nutrients that can be absorbed easily, worked as well as corticosteroids in producing remission in Crohn's disease.[7] However, the disease recurred when the patients returned to a normal diet,[7] thus indicating that something in the ordinary diet caused an immune response in Crohn's disease.[8]

Several studies have indicated that patients with Crohn's disease have an increased consumption of refined carbohydrates. In a four-year study conducted by Heaton, Thornton, and Emmett,[9] patients with Crohn's disease were instructed to follow a fiber-rich, unrefined-carbohydrate diet along with the usual forms of medicinal treatment. A comparison was made with thirty-two patients with Crohn's disease who did not receive any dietary instructions. Both hospital admissions and surgery were decreased in patients following the diet. This indicated that the reduction in consumption of refined carbohydrates may have favorably affected the health of patients with Crohn's disease.[9]

While the ingestion of carbohydrates may play a significant role, studies have also shown that sugar impacts Crohn's disease patients. A study done by Brandes and Lorenz-Meyer[10] examined the influence of a sugar-free diet on patients with Crohn's disease. Two groups of patients were treated with different diets. One group of ten patients followed a refined sugar-rich diet, and the other group of ten patients followed a sugar-free diet. In four of the ten patients who were given the sugar-rich diet, the study's treatment had to be discontinued due to increased disease activity. Decreased disease activity occurred in four of the ten patients who received the sugar-free diet throughout the study.[10]

Later, Brandes, Korst, and Littman[11] examined the influence of a sugar-free diet on twenty patients with Crohn's disease. These patients were receiving standard drug treatment when they began a sugar-free, fiber-rich diet. After remission was achieved, the drugs were discontinued, and the patients continued only the dietary treatment. Sixteen out of twenty patients remained in remission at the end of the twenty month study.[11] Thus, the impact of a sugar-free diet was evident.

When Mayberry, Rhodes, and Newcombe[12] interviewed 120 patients with Crohn's disease and 100 patients with ulcerative colitis and matched controls, the questionnaire revealed that patients with Crohn's disease consumed significantly more sugar than the patients with ulcerative colitis or the control group. Another interview was done by Reif and colleagues[13] with eighty-seven patients with ulcerative colitis and Crohn's disease, within one year after the onset of the illness, along with 144 healthy individuals. A reliable food analysis revealed that many patients with IBD consumed a higher amount of sucrose compared to the healthy people in the control group.[13]

These are just a few of the studies that have been done revealing the negative effects of an increased sugar diet on patients with Crohn's disease. This research leaves us to conclude that the consumption of sucrose affects the bacterial overgrowth seen in people with Crohn's disease. Greatly decreasing the amount of sucrose in the diet may favorably change the course of the disease.

Chapter 12

Friendly Bacteria

In the early 1900s, Elie Metchnikoff,[1] a Russian biologist and Nobel Prize winner for Medicine, described the observation that many long-living Bulgarians drank sour milk, a staple food in their diet. Microorganisms isolated from this milk contained a "very active lactic bacillus" which was named Bulgarian bacillus.[1] Metchnikoff noted that the microorganisms slowed down the growth of harmful intestinal bacteria. It was known then as Metchnikoff wrote, "There are many useful microbes, amongst which the lactic bacilli have an honourable place."[1] Although Metchnikoff received much criticism for his claims about the benefits of these bacteria, today, a hundred years later, research is escalating to further investigate the benefits of "friendly" bacteria. Much evidence indicates that they indeed have an "honourable place."

Since 1965, when Lilly and Stilwell first coined the term probiotic,[2] the definition has been revised several times. Fuller defined probiotics as "live microbial feed supplement which beneficially affects the host animal by improving its microbial balance."[3] Ingestion of these microorganisms has been shown to have a positive influence on health. Probiotics have the ability to compete with pathogens for nutrients, which the pathogens need to survive.[4]

Many probiotics are on the market today, but unless they are able to survive through the acids in the stomach to later reach the intestine, they are not of significant benefit. The specific strain called Lactobacillus GG has been the most widely studied of the probiotic agents, with over 250 clinical reports.[5] It was discovered in 1985 by Dr. Sherwood Gorbach and Dr. Barry Goldin of Tufts University and, therefore, was named Lactobacillus GG.[6] In their attempt to find this strain, they developed a list of ideal qualities for a lactobacillus strain they hoped to locate. They searched in the microflora of healthy humans for a strain that possessed their list of characteristics. "Thus, Lactobacillus GG was not manipulated, mutated, or altered in any way; it was found by natural selection."[6] Studies have shown encouraging results from administering Lactobacillus GG to patients with IBD.

In a six month study at the University of Chicago Children's hospital, children with Crohn's disease were given Lactobacillus GG at a dose of ten billion colony-forming units twice a day.[7] Patients showed significant improvement in the Crohn's disease activity within one week when measured by the pediatric Crohn's disease activity index (PCDAI). This index includes lab work, pain, diarrhea, and general well-being.[7]

Research has also indicated that some probiotics exhibit numerous benefits to the health of the intestinal tract, such as increased immunity, antibacterial effects, and ability to reduce allergies. Malin and colleages conducted a study in 1995 to determine immune responses of the antibody immunoglobulin A (IgA).[8] Fourteen children with Crohn's disease, nine with juvenile chronic arthritis, and seven in controls were given Lactobacillus GG for ten days.[8] Since IgA is known to prevent harmful bacteria and viruses "from invading the body through the mucosa of the gastrointestinal tract,"[9] a positive immune response was hypothesized. The results revealed increased antibody reactions, particularly in the children with Crohn's disease, indicating that Lactobacillus GG may be able to enhance the immunity of the intestinal tract.[8] By this action the protective barrier of cells on the intestinal wall becomes stronger, enabling it to fight against pathogens.[4]

We have observed Sarah's apparent increased immunity since she began following the sucrose-restricted diet and taking Culturelle®, which contains Lactobacillus GG. She has had only cold viruses with short durations in that time period. During her first month away at college, many students were sick with colds and coughs, but she was not. Her obviously improved immunity continues today, four years later.

In addition to increased immunity, probiotics have also been found to reduce allergies.[4] Further studies still need to be performed to understand the effects that probiotics have on the body's response to allergies; however, we have seen from first hand experience that they have clearly made a difference for Sarah in this aspect. Prior to her diagnosis of Crohn's disease, as mentioned earlier, she received allergy shots for allergies to dust, molds, and pollen. Sarah stopped receiving the injections due to the fevers they caused, but since taking Lactobacillus GG, her allergy symptoms have greatly reduced.

Thus, the benefits of probiotics are evident. From the research done on probiotics, particularly Lactobacillus GG, the results indicate that these "friendly" bacteria are capable of helping to restore good health for those suffering with Crohn's disease. Receiving a diagnosis in the early stages of this disorder and attempting to control its course through diet and probiotics may halt the disease for many people before it causes extensive damage.

Chapter 13

Enjoy Life

Sometimes, even though the complexities of an illness may not be understood, the solutions may be simple! A good example of this comes from the Bible story about a man named Naaman, who was a commander in the Syrian army. He was a great soldier, but he suffered from leprosy. When Naaman was sent to Elisha, the prophet, a messenger met him at the door telling him to go to the Jordan River, immerse himself seven times in the water, and receive healing. However, Naaman became angry. These instructions were not what Naaman expected, and he initially refused to obey. One of Naaman's servants then asked him if Elisha had instructed him to do something difficult, would he have done that? Naaman considered this and went to the Jordan

River. He immersed himself seven times as Elisha had ordered and was healed.

Many times when complex problems arise, I have been guilty of expecting a complicated solution, but sometimes there are simpler solutions. I remain grateful that Sarah's health has been restored by following the simple instructions of restricting sugar, eating plain yogurt, and taking Lactobacillus GG.

Dr. Poley once told Sarah as we were leaving his office, "Enjoy life." As a mom, I do not know of many things in life that have touched me more than to see my daughter continue to be healthy and enjoy life. My hope is that you also will be blessed with good health by simply following God's directions in whatever challenges you face. May you too enjoy life.

Chapter 14

Diet Guidelines

Many people live in the fast lane today, with minimal time to prepare foods that are healthy for meals, but even in the busyness of life, following this simple diet is manageable. Restricting the amount of sucrose (table sugar) as much as possible is the most important aspect of the diet Dr. Poley suggests. If you are one of many who suffer with a sugar addiction, realizing that craving for sweets typically decreases after restricting them for several weeks may be encouraging to you. An awareness of the naturally sweet taste of many foods becomes evident in time.

When Sarah began following the diet Dr. Poley recommends, we read labels of foods that she already frequently ate. Many items contained three grams or less of added sugar per serving, and this became our guideline.

In the recommended diet, the breads and starches allowed are crackers, bread, dinner rolls, pretzels, pancakes, waffles, cooked or dry cereals (without sugar coating), potatoes (white or sweet), pasta, and rice. These foods can generally be found with a minimal amount of sugar added to them. For example, numerous cereals contain one or two grams of sugar per serving, as do some sandwich breads and snack foods, such as crackers and pretzels. Varying amounts of sugar are frequently added to such foods as peanut butter, ketchup, salad dressings, and other processed foods, but it is possible to find ones (often available at natural foods stores) that do not have added sugar, only contain a minimal amount, or are sweetened with fruit.

All fresh, frozen, and canned vegetables without added sugar are allowed. It is especially important to read the labels of canned vegetables, since many have added sugar. Often with IBD, vegetables such as broccoli, kale, collards, cabbage, and cauliflower may cause extra gas, and whole kernel corn may be difficult to digest.

Fresh fruits and canned or frozen fruits without added sugar or syrup are allowed. Dried fruits are allowed but should be limited to eating occasionally or in small amounts since their sucrose content becomes higher in the drying stage. Fruit juices are not allowed, because they contain increased amounts of sucrose. Normally, many fruits contain some sucrose, but in juices, much fruit is needed to make a glass of juice, concentrating the sucrose level.

Meats allowed are beef, lamb, pork, veal, seafood, or poultry. Dried peas, beans, nuts, and peanut butter without added sugar are allowed.

Any kind of milk and yogurt without added sugar is allowed. If a lactose intolerance problem exists, lactose-free milk and cheeses without lactose are recommended. Since there is controversy over the effects of possible antibiotic residue in milk, organic dairy products may be preferable. Lactose-free yogurt can be made by using a yogurt machine and following the directions provided with the machine, but fermenting the yogurt for at least 24 hours to remove all of the lactose.

Soups without added sugar and combination foods, such as casseroles, that do not contain sweetened sauces or glazes are allowed.

Brown rice syrup, which contains mostly maltose, is allowed and can be found at natural foods stores. The sugar substitute Nutrasweet is allowed. Others should be avoided, such as lactitol, maltitol, sorbitol, xylitol, and mannitol, since they are incompletely absorbed from the intestine and may cause side effects of diarrhea. Sucralose and

Splenda are non-caloric sweeteners that are made from sugar cane and are not allowed. Honey, except in very minimal amounts, as well as molasses, pure maple syrup, and artificially flavored syrups, are not allowed due to their sucrose content.

Beverages that are allowed are water, tea, coffee, and sugar-free drinks with allowed sweeteners. Note that some people with Crohn's disease suffer from intestinal distress from drinking tap water, possibly due to chlorine content or other added irritants. Drinking distilled water or bottled water may be necessary, but be aware that some bottled waters with added minerals may also cause gastrointestinal distress.

Margarine, butter, vegetable oils, shortening, and salad dressings with limited sugar added are allowed. Cream and sour cream are allowed if not sensitive to lactose.

Condiments that are allowed are mustard, soy sauce, steak sauce, Worcestershire sauce, dill pickles, and ketchup without added sugar.

Sample menu

Breakfast: Cereal or egg and toast
1 serving of fruit
Water or milk

Lunch: Sandwich made with meat, cheese, or peanut butter

1 serving of fruit

1 or 2 servings of vegetables

Water or milk

Dinner: 2 choices of vegetables

Meat

Lettuce salad

1 serving of starch or grain, such as sweet potato, potato, rice, noodles, or roll

Water or milk

Snacks: Yogurt, fruit, pretzels, crackers

Note about our experience with Culturelle®:

We noted that Sarah tolerated best the type of Culturelle® product that contains inulin along with the Lactobacillus GG. When she first started taking the Culturelle® capsule, she began with ½ of a capsule, which we added to applesauce, and then she gradually increased the dose to 2 capsules per day after approximately a ten-day time span, taking 1 capsule in the morning and 1 capsule at dinner time. It may cause extra gas while the gastrointestinal tract adjusts to having much more "good" bacteria enter it, but gas should subside within two weeks.

Recipes

Tips about Recipes

Included are some sample recipes of entrees, vegetables, breads, and cookies that we enjoy. Of course, moderation of desserts would be wise.

Many of your own favorite recipes can be utilized by simply using ingredients that contain minimal or no amounts of sucrose.

Rice syrup can be found in many natural foods stores. It can be substituted in recipes as an equal replacement for table sugar.

Fructose crystals contain some sucrose, and it is best to use them sparingly. They can be mixed easily with cinnamon, poured into a shaker, and sprinkled lightly on foods such as muffins, cookies, or sweet potatoes.

Chicken and Vegetables Stir-Fry

2 tablespoons olive oil

½ cup sliced celery

1 cup water

2 cups diced, cooked chicken

2 cups cooked rice

4 cups frozen mixed vegetables, partially thawed

1–2 tablespoons soy sauce

Heat oil in a skillet or wok. Add celery. Stir-fry for 1 minute. Add water and bring to a boil. Add chicken, rice, and vegetables. Stir in soy sauce. Cover and cook for 5 minutes, stirring occasionally, until vegetables are at desired tenderness.

Makes 4–6 servings.

Chicken Salad

2 cups diced, cooked chicken

½ cup mayonnaise

⅔ cup sliced grapes

½ cup chopped pecans

¼ teaspoon curry powder

Mix chicken, grapes, and pecans together. Combine mayonnaise and curry powder. Add mayonnaise and curry powder mixture to chicken mixture.

Makes 4 servings.

Tuna Quiche

1 9 - inch pie shell

12 ½ oz. can of tuna (drained)

½ cup shredded Swiss cheese

3 eggs

½ cup mayonnaise

½ cup milk

Chopped onion, if desired

Pierce pastry with fork. Bake in 375-degree oven for 10 minutes. Remove from oven.

In large bowl, mix together tuna, cheese, and eggs. Spoon into pie shell.

In bowl, mix together mayonnaise and milk. Slowly pour this over tuna mixture.

Bake at 350 degrees for 45–50 minutes or until center comes out clean with knife.

Makes 6 servings.

Chicken Pot Pie

1 9 - inch pie crust

2 cups mixed vegetables

2 cups diced, cooked chicken

½ teaspoon thyme

½ teaspoon pepper

1 cup chicken bouillon

2 tablespoons butter or margarine

2 tablespoons flour

Combine vegetables and chicken in pie dish.

In sauce pan, melt butter and stir in flour. Add bouillon, thyme, and pepper. Stir until thick like gravy. Pour over chicken and vegetable mixture. Top with the pie crust, and prick crust with fork.

Bake at 350 degrees for 45 minutes.

Makes 4–6 servings.

Meatloaf

1 pound ground beef
1 egg, slightly beaten
¼ cup unsweetened ketchup
½ cup crushed soda crackers
Chopped onion, if desired

In bowl, combine hamburger, egg, and ketchup. Mix together well. Place mixture in small loaf pan.

Bake at 350 degrees for 30 minutes, then sprinkle cracker crumbs on top and bake 10 more minutes.

Makes 4 servings.

Lasagna (Lactose free)

1 pound ground beef

1 can (15 oz.) tomato sauce without added sugar—add seasoning of onion and garlic, if desired

1 package (8 oz.) lasagna noodles, cooked and drained

8 oz. sharp cheddar cheese, shredded

8 oz. lactose-free cottage cheese

Cook ground beef in skillet, drain off fat.

Add tomato sauce and season as desired.

Simmer for 5 minutes.

Place 3 pieces of lasagna noodles on bottom of 13 x 9 - inch baking dish.

Spread 1/3 of sauce over noodles.

Spread ½ container cottage cheese over sauce.

Sprinkle 1/3 of cheddar cheese over cottage cheese.

Repeat 2nd layer of noodles, 1/3 of sauce and remaining cottage cheese, and 1/3 cheddar cheese.

Place 3rd layer of noodles, and top with remaining sauce and cheddar cheese.

Bake at 350 degrees for 30–40 minutes.

Makes 8–10 servings.

Sweet Potato Casserole

4 medium sweet potatoes, cooked and peeled

1 egg

¼ cup orange juice

¼ cup plus 2 tablespoons melted butter or margarine

1 teaspoon salt

1 teaspoon cinnamon

2 teaspoons fructose crystals

½ cup pecan halves

Mash sweet potatoes with fork and place in large bowl. Add egg, orange juice, and ¼ cup melted butter or margarine to sweet potatoes. Beat until light and fluffy. Pour into baking dish.

Arrange pecan halves on sweet potato mixture.

Mix cinnamon and fructose crystals with the remaining melted butter or margarine. Drizzle over casserole.

Bake at 350 degrees for 30 minutes.

Serves 4–6.

Spaghetti Squash

Prick holes in squash with sharp knife.

For small size squash, bake for 5 minutes on high in microwave and then turn to bake on opposite side for 5 minutes.

Cut squash in half length-wise, scoop out center portion of seeds. With fork, pull strings of squash out from center. If not tender, place open sides of cut halves on dish and cook additional minutes until squash scoops out easily.

Top with butter or tomato sauce.

Serves 4–6.

Pumpkin Bread

1 cup oil

1 ½ cups brown rice syrup

3 eggs

2 cups pumpkin (1-lb. can)

3 ½ cups flour

½ teaspoon baking powder

2 teaspoons baking soda

1 teaspoon salt

1 teaspoon cinnamon

½ teaspoon each allspice, nutmeg

¼ teaspoon cloves

1 cup chopped nuts and raisins, if desired

Mix oil and brown rice syrup together. Beat in eggs. Mix in pumpkin.

Add flour, baking powder, baking soda, salt, cinnamon, allspice, nutmeg, and cloves to pumpkin mixture. Blend in nuts and raisins if desired. Pour mixture into 2 loaf pans.

Bake at 350 degrees for 45–55 minutes or until knife comes out clean.

Muffins

1 egg
4 tablespoons melted butter
1 cup milk
¼ cup rice syrup
2 cups all-purpose flour or a mixture of whole wheat and white flour
3 teaspoons baking powder
½ teaspoon salt

Lightly beat egg and mix with milk, butter, and rice syrup.

Add remaining ingredients and stir until batter is moistened.

Fill greased muffin pans until 2/3 full.

Bake at 350 degrees for 15 minutes. Makes 12 muffins.

Variation: Stir in one cup blueberries to batter, if desired.

Blueberry Cobbler with Oatmeal Crust

3 cups fresh or frozen blueberries

½ teaspoon cinnamon

¾ cup oat flour or all-purpose flour

1 cup oats

½ cup butter

¼ cup rice syrup

Stir cinnamon with blueberries and pour into 9-inch pie plate.

Mix remaining ingredients together and spread over blueberries.

Bake at 350 degrees for 30–40 minutes or until crust is done.

Makes 6 servings.

Apple Pie

2 9 - inch pie crusts

4 cups sliced, pared apples

½ teaspoon cinnamon

1 teaspoon fructose crystals

Mix apples, cinnamon, and fructose crystals together and arrange mixture in pie crust. Top with the second crust; make slits in crust with knife.

Bake at 350 degrees for 45 minutes.

Makes 6–8 servings.

Chocolate Chip Cookies

½ cup brown rice syrup

½ cup (1 stick) softened butter

½ teaspoon vanilla

1 egg

1 cup plus 4 tablespoons flour

½ teaspoon baking soda

½ teaspoon salt

½ cup grain-sweetened chocolate chips

Chopped pecans or walnuts if desired

Mix first 4 ingredients together and beat until blended. Add flour, soda, and salt to mixture, and beat together. Add grain-sweetened chocolate chips. Add nuts if desired.

Bake at 350 degrees for 10 to 12 minutes.

Makes about 2 dozen cookies.

Butter Cookies

¾ cup softened butter

½ cup brown rice syrup

¾ teaspoon vanilla

1⅔ cup flour

½ teaspoon salt

Cinnamon mixed with fructose crystals

Mix butter, brown rice syrup, and vanilla together until creamy. Add flour and salt to mixture, and blend well. Chill dough until firm. Shape dough into balls. Flatten with bottom of glass OR roll out dough and cut with cookie cutters. Sprinkle cookies with cinnamon fructose crystals. Bake at 350 degrees for 10 minutes.

Makes about 2 dozen cookies.

Endnotes

Chapter 9

1. Beaumont, W. (1833). *Experiments and observation on the gastric juice and physiology of digestion.* New York: Peter Smith, 1941. (Facsimile of the original edition of 1833.)

Chapter 11

1. Wilson, K. (1995). Gastrointestinal Microflora. T. Yamada (Ed.), *Textbook of gastroenterolgy.* (2nd ed., pp. 609–615). Philadelphia: JB Lippincott.

2. Moore, W. E. C., & Holdeman, L. V. (1974). Human fecal flora: The normal flora of 20

Japanese-Hawaiians. *Applied Microbiology, 27*(5), 961–979.

3. Madsen, K., Cornish, A., Soper, P., McKaigney, C., Jijon, H., Yachimec, C., et al. (2001). Probiotic bacteria enhance murine and human intestinal epithelial barrier function. *Gastroenterology, 121*, 580–591.

4. Hart, A. L., Stagg, A. J., & Kamm, M. A. (2003). Use of probiotics in the treatment of inflammatory bowel disease. *Journal of Clinical Gastroenterology, 36*(2), 111–117.

5. Hugot, J. P., Zouali, H., & Lesage, S. (2003). Lessons to be learned from NOD2 gene in Crohn's disease. *European Journal of Gastroenterology and Hepatology, 15*(6), 593–7.

6. Poley, J. R. (1983). Chronic nonspecific diarrhea in children: investigation of surface morphology of small bowel mucosa utilizing the scanning electron microscope. *Journal of Pediatric Gastroenterology and Nutrition, 2*(1), 71–94.

7. Ó'Moráin, C., Segal, A. W., & Levi, A. J. (1984). Elemental diet as primary treatment of acute Crohn's disease: a controlled trial. *British Medical Journal, 288*, 1859–62.

8. Mahmud, N., & Weir, D. G. (2001). The urban diet and Crohn's disease: is there a relationship?

European Journal of Gastroenterology and Hepatology, 13(2), 93–95.

9. Heaton, K. W., Thornton, J. R., & Emmett, P. M. (1979). Treatment of Crohn's disease with an unrefined-carbohydrate, fibre-rich diet. *British Medical Journal, 2*, 764–766.

10. Brandes, J. W., & Lorenz-Meyer, H. (1981). Sugar-free diet: a new perspective in the treatment of Crohn's disease? Randomized control study. [Abstract]. *Z Gastroenterology, 19*(1), 1–12.

11. Brandes, J. W., Korst, H. A., & Littman, K. P. (1982). Sugar-free diet as long-term or interval treatment in the remission phase of Crohn's disease—a prospective study. [Abstract]. *Leber Magen Darm, 12*(6), 225–8.

12. Mayberry, J. F., Rhodes, J., & Newcombe, R. G. (1980). Increased sugar consumption in Crohn's Disease. *Digestion, 20*, 323–326.

13. Reif, S., Klein, I., Lubin, F., Farbstein, M., Hallak, A., & Gilat, T. (1997). Pre-illness dietary factors in inflammatory bowel disease. *GUT, 40*, 754–760.

Chapter 12

1. Metchnikoff, E. (1908). *The prolongation of life: optimistic studies.* New York and London: G.P. Putnam's Sons.

2. Lilly, D., & Stillwell, R. (1965). Probiotics: growth-promoting factors produced by microorgansims. *Science, 147,* 747–748.
3. Fuller, R. (1991). Probiotics in human medicine. *Gut, 32,* 439–442.
4. Michail, S. (2005). The mechanism of action of probiotics. *Practical gastroenterology,* 29–47.
5. Amerifit Brands. (2007). *Answering your questions about Culturelle®* [Pamphlet]. Cromwell, CT: Amerifit Brands, Inc.
6. Gorbach, S. (2000). Probiotics and gastrointestinal health. *The American Journal of Gastroenterology, 95,* (suppl.): S2–S3.
7. Gupta, P., Andrew, H., Kirschner, B. S., & Guandalini, S. (2000). Is Lactobacillus GG helpful in children with Crohn's disease? Results of a preliminary, open-label study. *Journal of Pediatric Gastroenterology Nutrition, 31*(4), 453–7.
8. Malin, M., Suomalainen, H., Saxelin, M., & Isolauri, E. (1996). Promotion of IgA immune response in patients with Crohn's disease by oral bacteriotherapy with Lactobacillus GG. *Annals of Nutrition and Metabolism, 40*(3), 137–45.
9. Venes, Donald, (Ed.), (2001). *Taber's cyclopedic medical dictionary.* Philadelphia: F. A. Davis Company.

References

Amerifit Brands. (2007). *Answering your questions about Culturelle®* [Pamphlet]. Cromwell, CT: Amerifit Brands, Inc.

Beaumont, W. (1833). *Experiments and observation on the gastric juice and physiology of digestion.* New York: Peter Smith, 1941. (Facsimile of the original edition of 1833.)

Brandes, J. W., Korst, H. A., & Littman, K. P. (1982). Sugar-free diet as long term or interval treatment in the remission phase of Crohn's disease—a prospective study. [Abstract]. *Leber Magen Darm, 12*(6), 225–8.

Brandes, J. W., & Lorenz-Meyer, H. (1981). Sugar-free diet: a new perspective in the treatment of

Crohn's disease? Randomized control study. [Abstract]. *Z Gastroenterology, 19*(1), 1–12.

Fuller, R. (1991). Probiotics in human medicine. *Gut, 32,* 439–442.

Gorbach, S. (2000). Probiotics and gastrointestinal health. *The American Journal of Gastroenterology, 95,* (suppl.): S2–S3.

Gupta, P., Andrew, H., Kirschner, B. S., & Guandalini, S. (2000). Is Lactobacillus GG helpful in children with Crohn's disease? Results of a preliminary, open-label study. *Journal of Pediatric Gastroenterology Nutrition, 31*(4), 453–7.

Hart, A. L., Stagg, A. J., & Kamm, M. A. (2003). Use of probiotics in the treatment of inflammatory bowel disease. *Journal of Clinical Gastorenterology, 36*(2), 111–117.

Heaton, K. W., Thornton, J. R., & Emmett, P. M. (1979). Treatment of Crohn's disease with an unrefined-carbohydrate, fibre-rich diet. *British Medical Journal, 2,* 764–766.

Hugot, J. P., Zouali, H., & Lesage, S. (2003). Lessons to be learned from NOD2 gene in Crohn's disease. *European Journal of Gastroenterology and Hepatology, 15*(6), 593–7.

Lilly, D., & Stillwell, R. (1965). Probiotics: growth promoting factors produced by microorgansims. *Science, 147,* 747–748.

Madsen, K., Cornish, A., Soper, P., McKaigney, C., Jijon, H., Yachimec, C., et al. (2001). Probiotic bacteria enhance murine and human intestinal epithelial barrier function. *Gastroenterology, 121,* 580–591.

Mahmud, N., & Weir, D. G. (2001). The urban diet and Crohn's disease: is there a relationship? *European Journal of Gastroenterology and Hepatology, 13*(2), 93–95.

Malin, M., Suomalainen, H., Saxelin, M., & Isolauri, E. (1996). Promotion of IgA immune response in patients with Crohn's disease by oral bacteriotherapy with Lactobacillus GG. *Annals of Nutrition and Metabolism, 40*(3), 137–45.

Mayberry, J. F., Rhodes, J., & Newcombe, R.G. (1980). Increased sugar consumption in Crohn's disease. *Digestion, 20,* 323–326.

Metchnikoff, E. (1908). *The prolongation of life: optimistic studies.* New York: G.P. Putnam's Sons.

Michail, S. (2005). The mechanism of action of probiotics. *Practical Gastroenterology,* 29–47.

Moore, W. E. C., & Holdeman, L.V. (1974). Human fecal flora: The normal flora of 20 Japanese-Hawaiians, *Applied Microbiology, 27*(5), 961–979.

Ó'Moráin, C., Segal, A. W., & Levi, A. J. (1984). Elemental diet as primary treatment of acute Crohn's disease: a controlled trial. *British Medical Journal, 288*, 1859–62.

Poley, J. R. (1983). Chronic nonspecific diarrhea in children: investigation of surface morphology of small bowel mucosa utilizing the scanning electron microscope. *Journal of Pediatric Gastroenterology and Nutrition, 2*(1), 71–94.

Reif, S., Klein, I., Lubin, F., Farbstein, M., Hallak, A., & Gilat, T. (1997). Pre-illness dietary factors in inflammatory bowel disease. *GUT, 40*, 754–760.

Venes, Donald, (Ed.), (2001). *Taber's cyclopedic medical dictionary.* Philadelphia: F. A. Davis Company.

Wilson, K. (1995). Gastrointestinal Microflora. T. Yamada, (Ed.), *Textbook of gastroenterology.* (2nd ed., pp. 609–615). Philadelphia: JB Lippincott.

To order additional copies of this title:
Please visit our Web site at
www.pleasantwordbooks.com

If you enjoyed this quality custom-published book,
drop by our Web site for more books and information.

www.winepressgroup.com
"Your partner in custom publishing."